Marija Knežević-Pogančev
Nebojša Jović
Gorana Pogančev

Disposition factors and specific trigger of migraine headache in adole

AF144443

Marija Knežević-Pogančev
Nebojša Jović
Gorana Pogančev

Disposition factors and specific trigger of migraine headache in adole

Migraine headache in adolescents

LAP LAMBERT Academic Publishing

Impressum / Imprint
Bibliografische Information der Deutschen Nationalbibliothek: Die Deutsche Nationalbibliothek verzeichnet diese Publikation in der Deutschen Nationalbibliografie; detaillierte bibliografische Daten sind im Internet über http://dnb.d-nb.de abrufbar.
Alle in diesem Buch genannten Marken und Produktnamen unterliegen warenzeichen-, marken- oder patentrechtlichem Schutz bzw. sind Warenzeichen oder eingetragene Warenzeichen der jeweiligen Inhaber. Die Wiedergabe von Marken, Produktnamen, Gebrauchsnamen, Handelsnamen, Warenbezeichnungen u.s.w. in diesem Werk berechtigt auch ohne besondere Kennzeichnung nicht zu der Annahme, dass solche Namen im Sinne der Warenzeichen- und Markenschutzgesetzgebung als frei zu betrachten wären und daher von jedermann benutzt werden dürften.

Bibliographic information published by the Deutsche Nationalbibliothek: The Deutsche Nationalbibliothek lists this publication in the Deutsche Nationalbibliografie; detailed bibliographic data are available in the Internet at http://dnb.d-nb.de.
Any brand names and product names mentioned in this book are subject to trademark, brand or patent protection and are trademarks or registered trademarks of their respective holders. The use of brand names, product names, common names, trade names, product descriptions etc. even without a particular marking in this work is in no way to be construed to mean that such names may be regarded as unrestricted in respect of trademark and brand protection legislation and could thus be used by anyone.

Coverbild / Cover image: www.ingimage.com

Verlag / Publisher:
LAP LAMBERT Academic Publishing
ist ein Imprint der / is a trademark of
OmniScriptum GmbH & Co. KG
Heinrich-Böcking-Str. 6-8, 66121 Saarbrücken, Deutschland / Germany
Email: info@lap-publishing.com

Herstellung: siehe letzte Seite /
Printed at: see last page
ISBN: 978-3-659-48828-3

Copyright © 2015 OmniScriptum GmbH & Co. KG
Alle Rechte vorbehalten. / All rights reserved. Saarbrücken 2015

To our patients suffering headache

Contents

Abstract

Disposition factors, as a factor of risk for migraine headache do not directly neither cause migraine headache. Trigger factors are provoking migraine headache in for migraine headache predisponded adolescents. Recognizing specific age dependent migraine headache disposition and trigger factors in adolescents, some of migraine headaches can be avoided.

Study was conducted on 20,917 adolescents in Serbia.

Apparently from a direct heredity, as adolescents migraine headache disposition factors should also be accepted: the order of birth, the length of breast-feeding, age when the ready-made industrial food was introduced, age when the child was introduced to a whole-day basis stay, kinetosis and insufficient dominance of the hemisphere. Migraine headache trigger factors in adolescents are specific and age dependent. Typical migraine headache trigger factors in adolescents are lack of sleep, tobacco passive smoking, alcohol intakes, and "not eating at time".

Identification of migraine headache trigger factors is extremely important especially in adolescents with clear migraine headache disposition factors. Their elimination directly provides prevention of migraine headaches in adolescents.

By avoiding specific trigger factors, in more than half of adolescent's reduction of drug use in headache therapy can be achieved.

Adolescence

Adolescence (adolescere (Latin) "to grow up") is defined as a transitional stage of physical and psychological human development period between puberty and adulthood, closely associated with the teenage years (1). Generally adolescence occurs during the period from puberty to legal adulthood extending mainly over the teen years and terminating legally when the age of majority is reached youth (2). A thorough understanding of adolescence in society depends on information from various perspectives, including psychology, biology, physiology, history, sociology, education, and anthropology.

From social aspect adolescence is a period or stage of cognitive development, and society, preceding maturity. From medical aspect adolescence is the process or state of growing to maturity. Adolescence can be defined:

- **biologically,** as the physical transition marked by the onset of puberty and the termination of physical growth;

- **cognitively,** as changes in the ability to think abstractly and multi-dimensionally;

- **socially,** as a period of preparation for adult roles.

Adolescence may be roughly divided into three stages:

- **early adolescence,** ages eleven to fourteen;

- **middle adolescence,** ages fifteen to seventeen;

- **late adolescence**, ages eighteen to twenty-one.

In addition to physiological growth, intellectual, psychological and social developmental tasks are squeezed into these years. Adolescence is a period of multiple transitions involving education, training, and transitions from one living circumstance to another. Thus chronological age provides only a rough marker of adolescence, with lot of difficulties upon a precise definition (3, 4, 5).

Migraine headache

Migraine headache, as a form of a headache, was described even 5000 years ago in a Sumerian poem of "Dilhum – a paradise on the Earth". Eber papyrus, 3500 years ago, tells about the illness of one of the hemisphere of the head. Egyptian manuscripts dating from 1500 years B.C. tell about the migraine headache (6). Aretheus from Cappadocia, in the 1st century A.D. called the migraine headache "heterocranios", and described it as a paroxysmal, unilateral pain in the head, followed by nausea and vomiting repeated in regular time intervals. In the 2nd century A.D. Galen uses the term "hemicranios", thus explaining the nausea and vomiting as being the result of the activity of toxic wastes caused by secretion in organs suffering disorders (6). The term was taken over by the Romans as "hemicrania" who pronounced it as "hemigranea", the origin of the current name – migraine. Hippocrtates knowledge on migraine headache echoed in the treatment of all those who suffered headaches in the first Serbian hospital in Hilandar in 1197, and Studenica from 1206-1217. Migraine headaches were also the issue in the Hospital of King Milutin in Constantinople, in 1308, with Jovan Argiropulos as a head. Unfortunately, neither the "Codex 517" nor the other written monuments of our medical culture recorded this suffering in piece and silence (6).

Migraine headache, as an entity, is not fully understood, because it lacks clear laboratory correlations and objective defining markers. No anatomical changes are known to represent the basis of migraine headache. In the opinion of a great number of authors today, migraine headache, as a very complex syndrome, is still a matter of deduction (7). There is not enough knowledge on signs and symptoms or on personal and family anamnesis of adolescents with migraine headaches, to clearly distinguish all clinical entities of migraine headache during developmental age. Symptoms of migraine headache attacks are most important in identification of migraine headache in adults. Different criteria are suggested as diagnostic criteria of migraine headache in children, preadolescents and adolescents (8, 9).

Migraine headache is a chronic neurological disorder characterized by episodic attacks of headaches with different intensity, frequency and duration, commonly unilateral and associated with anorexia, nausea, vomiting, photo- and phonophobia. Some are preceded or accompanied by sensory, motor or affective changes. Sensory, vegetative, affective and various combinations of neurological, gastrointestinal and vegetative migraine headache phenomena are found only in humans. The degree of their expression varies, both qualitatively and quantitatively from patient to patient (10).

The migraine headache syndrome as a striking example of interdisciplinary, health, practical and clinical entity, represents a current problem in adolescent neurology even today, and the degree of interest is in a direct proportion to the level of social and health standard in the society (11).

Migraine headache in adolescents

Headache disorders are remarkably common in adolescents (12, 13, 14).

Migraine headache is the primary type of headache in adolescence (15). Adolescents' migraine headache is a chronic neurological disorder mostly characterized by episodic attacks of headaches with different intensity, frequency and duration, commonly unilateral and associated with anorexia, nausea, vomiting, phono- and photophobia. Very often preceded or accompanied by sensory, motor, vegetative, affective and various combinations of neurological, gastrointestinal and vegetative changes. The degree of their qualitatively and quantitatively expression vary in adolescents (16). According to the literature data, generally, pain quality and localization, attacks duration, behavioral markers accompanying symptoms and remission occurrence rate seem to be age dependent (17, 18).

Migraine headache diagnosis

Migraine headache diagnosis depends on systematic secondary disorders exclusion and systematic specific features of the primary disorders identification. Adolescent's migraine headache, as a very complex syndrome, is still a matter of deduction. It seems to be a complex disorder caused by influence of multiple genes and environmental factors (19). Exact cause of migraine headache is unknown. There are no laboratory based diagnostic tests to identify acute migraine headache attack, as well as no tests to recognize migraine headache sufferers (20). There is not enough knowledge of age dependent specific signs and symptoms, to clearly distinguish all clinical entities of adolescent migraine headache. It is largely underestimated and misdiagnosed, because of the lack of anatomical changes, specific biological markers and specific research tools or brain imaging techniques. Migraine headache phenomena: sensory, vegetative and affective, found only in humans, with marked age dependent quantitative and qualitative variations which differ from adolescent to adolescent, are outlining the adolescent migraine headache. In the opinion of a great number of authors today, adolescent migraine headache, as a very complex syndrome, is still a matter of deduction (16). According to Barlow's definition, migraine headache reflects an inherited vulnerability and vasomotor instability (8). Family and twin studies show that there is a genetic component to migraine headache, but no genes predisposing to common forms of the disorder have been identified, and the actual types of responsible genes are still not fully understood (21). No empirical study has explicitly examined how genetic and environmental factors influence the adolescent's migraine headache (22, 23).

Generally speaking, it is hard to define type of adolescent headache, particularly migraine headaches. In the opinion of a great number of authors today, very complex syndrome of adolescent migraine headache is still a matter of deduction. Different classification and diagnostic migraine headache criteria are suggested in adolescents (24).

Vahlquist in 1955. gave diagnostic criteria for children migraine headache (25). In 1962. Rother published a classification of children's headaches based on the time pattern. Migraine headache classifications were also given by Bille in 1962, Prensky in 1976, Debner in 1977, Congdon and Forsythe in 1979, Tomasi in 1980, Sillanappa in 1982, Kurtz and Barlow in 1984, Hockaday in 1988 (26, 27, 28, 29, 30, 31, 32).

Instead of "diagnostic and classification criteria for headaches, cranial neuralgia and facial pain", from International Association for Headaches (IHS) from 1988, and ICHD-II (International Classification of Headache Disorders) from September 2003. what is officially used today is The International Classification of Headache Disorders 3rd edition (beta version) (33).

Exact cause of migraine headache is unknown. There are no laboratory based diagnostic tests to identify those who suffer from the disorder. The mechanisms underlying migraine headache are largely unknown. Many migraine headache sufferers have a family history of migraine headache but the exact hereditary nature of migraine headaches is still being determined. They seem to be a complex disorder caused by influence of multiple genes and environmental factors Family and twin studies show that there is a genetic component to migraine headache, but no genes predisposing to common forms of the disorder have been identified (34). Genetic disposition of the migraine headache is certainly present, but the path of genetic transmission is still neither clear nor completely comprehensible. Goodell and Wolf in 1954. wrote about the somatic recessive heredity, Barolin and Linet in 1991. wrote about the dominant heredity with higher probability of penetration among women, and Douglas-Nielsen about poly-genetic heredity (35, 36).

The modern genetic hereditary concept suggests multifactor heredity in which several genes take place. Hemiplegic family migraine headache is, for the time being, the only migraine headache type with potential genetic marker (37).

There is a very high degree of mutual dependence between the migraine headache of the twin siblings shown through correlation and determination quotient of the migraine headache. Higher dependence and importance of the difference with monozygotic twins confirm the hereditability of the migraine headache, migraine with aura in particular (38). The modern genetic heredity concept suggests migraine headache multifactor heredity in which several genes takes place (39).

Migraine headache disposition factors

Migraine headache disposition factors do not represent the factors of risk at the same time, they do not directly cause migraine headache, nor have the clear causative relation to the migraine headache. Disposition factors recognized in adolescent's predisposed to migraine headache do not represent the factors of risk at the same time, they do not directly cause migraine headache, nor have the clear causative relation to the migraine headache. Different single-variant or multi-variant analyses recognize them in personality traits, social milieu, intelligence, relation to the surroundings, working ability and activity, and in the very personal approach to illness itself.

Many different studies dealing with adolescents who suffer from the migraine headache, stress the behavioral disorder in the form of perfectionism. They describe the adolescents as being sensitive, active, nervous, and too caring and conscientious from the earliest childhood. They are often frightened, emotionally shaped by their parents, with high depressive, anxiety and psychosomatic disorder score (40).

Hormonal factors are at the same time basic, constitutional, dispositional, but also a precipitating factor of the migraine headache. Distribution of the migraine headache with and without aura according to the gender is different. However, the influence of gender-dependent factors is more striking with migraine headache without aura (41).

The hypothesis about a low basic level of monoamine oxidize and noradrenergic malfunction, explains the fact that a large number of factors (stress, hormones and tyramine) can trigger the migraine headache attack (over-constriction of cerebral arteries) (42).

No precise literature data and differentiated standpoints about the dominance of hemispheres in adolescent migraine headache can be found. Knežević-Pogančev described in 2004th in a group of left-handed children the migraine headache present among 2.3% of them, non-migraine headaches among 33.1% of them. In a group of right-handed children Knežević-Pogančev reported the migraine headache present among 7.8% children, non-migraine headache among 18.2% of them. In the group of children with insufficient dominance of the hemisphere Knežević-Pogančev reported 18.6% children had migraine headaches and 14.9% non-migraine headaches (10).

Among the children having migraine headache 1.8% was left-handed, 73.8% right-handed, and even 24.4% of them vere children with insufficient dominance of the hemisphere. Autor proved lower presence of both left-handed and right-handed children with a significant higher presence in children with insufficient dominance of the hemisphere within the group of children with the migraine headache, proving clear relation between the dominance of the hemisphere and migraine headache (10).

There are no literature data proving breastfeeding influence of migraine headache except our group paper published in 2012. (43). Knežević-Pogančev and coautors wrote about influence of breastfeeding duration on the manifestation of migraine headache and age at onset of migraine headache symptoms. They show reslts by analyzing history data on headache of 30,636 children aged 3-17 residing in Vojvodina and on nutrition in 24,011 of these subjects. Data were compared between children with migraine headache (8.63%) and other primary recurrent headaches (18.83%). Negative Pearson correlation ratio (0.07, p<0.01) clearly showed reciprocal influence of the duration of breastfeeding on the migraine headache onset and earlier onset of migraine in children who were breastfed for a shorter time (p<0.01). Autors concluded that defining the duration of breastfeeding as an early predisposing factor for migraine headache offers the possibility of very early migraine headache prevention, especially in children with positive heredity for migraine headache (43).

Sillanapaa and associates suggest that the following factors are the cause for the appearance of migraine headache: poor economic status of the family, child`s stay at the nursery school (a whole-day stay), a great number of school activities, especially within the group of children where a headache appeared before 5 years of age.

All analyzed risk disposition factors are nonspecific for headache in adolescents because they also increase the risk for other health complaints. Diagnostic procedure and intervention therefore, should consider a holistic approach focusing not only on headache but also on a broader spectrum of health complaints (44).

Migraine headache underlying mechanism

According to Barlow's definition, migraine headache reflects an inherited vulnerability and vasomotor instability, and trigger factors are exclusive occurrences which decompensate the nervous system (8). From Galen onwards, to the 18th century, there are no written scientific descriptions of the migraine headache. By analyzing his own headache, Lepois in 1714, indicates that meteorological factors have a provocative role in triggering migraine headaches. Lewis described his own visual hallucinations when writing "Alice in Wonderland". Vater and Heinicke described the ophthalmophlegic migraine headache in 1723, and a year later, Anhalt discussed the vascular component in etiology of the migraine headache pain. Fothergili in 1773. described the neuralgic facial pain. Tissoti in 1783. gave the importance to gastrointestinal disorders in origin of migraine headache seizures, explaining the activity of the nervous stimuli from the abdomen directly on the brain. Piorry in 1835. described the scintillating scotoma of the migraine headache aura and their vascular etiology. Trousseau, Charcot and Lasegue supplemented these observations. Raymond in 1860. concludes that the migraine headache is a "vasomotor neurosis", which comes as a consequence of an irritation of the cervical sympathetic nerves. Molendorf assumes that the paralysis of the sympathetic nervous system is due to a vascular component.

Wolf and the associates (Friedman, Ostfield, Tunis, Delessio, Sicuteri, Graham) from 1937. to 1959. confirmed the causal relation between the migraine headache and transitory dysfunction of arterial and capillary cranial blood vessels. They supplemented the "Mechanical" theory of the migraine headache with a hypothesis of the transudation of "neurosis" in a phase of dilatation from plasma into the perivascular tissue. Sicuteri in 1958. explained the etiology of migraine headache by systematic disorders in metabolism of vasoneuroactive substances. Chapman in 1960. identified the "neurocin" whose presence in the region of trigeminal of experimental animals is documented by Moskowitz in 1979 . Serotonine theory is accepted by Curran in 1965, Anthony and Lance in 1971, Rydzewicki in 1976, Delessio in 1976, and Muck-Seler in 1979. Thrombocytal serotonin and hyperaggregability of the thrombocytes in pathophysiology of the migraine headache were defined by Hilton and Cumings in 1972, Kalendovsky and Austin in 1975, Couch and Hassanein, Deshunk and Mayer in 1977, Jones and D`Andrea and associates in 1982 .

Curran in 1965, Rydzewicki in 1976, Delessio in 1976, Hardebo in 1978, Muck-Seler in 1979, Fozard in 1990, Moskowitz in 1993, Silberstein in 1994 defined the vasomotoric effect of the serotonine 5 - hydroxytryptamine (5HT) during the migraine seizure, recording the increase of 5-hydroxy-indoleacetic acid in urine. Gaddum and Picarelli in 1957. found out two 5HT receptors, and Peroutka and Snyder set up the basis for a modern classification of receptors 5HT. Leao in 1944. defined the phenomenon of a "spreading depression of the electrical activity" - a wave of visible dilatation, joined together with a peak of electrophysiological depression that, 45 years later, Welsh managed to visualize electromagnetically during the migraine headache attack. Milner in 1958. discussed the similarity between the progression of scotoma in the migraine headache aura and Leao's spreading depression.

Cervicocephalus syndrome as a clinical entity was interpreted by Schytzenberger and Lieou in 1853. In 1925. Barre gave a detailed description, and Bartch-Rochaix called it "migraine cervicale" in 1949. Strumpell was the first one to recognize the allergic factors in etiology of a headache in 1883. In 1927. Waugham described allergic headaches and Reader allergic migraine headache form in 1924. Friedman described post-traumatic headaches, Breuer and Freud defined psychogenesis, and Mathew combined headaches in 1981. In 1926. Harris described a Cluster headache as the "periodical migraine like neuralgia". In 1941. Horton introduced the term "histaminic headache".

Exact cause of migraine headache is unknown. There are no laboratory based diagnostic tests to identify those who suffer from the disorder. The mechanisms underlying migraine headache are largely unknown. They seem to be a complex disorder caused by influence of multiple genes and environmental factors (45, 46).

Most of authors take the positive family anamnesis to be one of the diagnostic criteria of the migraine headache. Many migraine headache sufferers have a family history of migraine headache but the exact hereditary nature of migraines headache is still being determined. Positive family data of the recurrent headaches was detected among 98.6% children with migraine headaches, 64.7% children with non-migraine headaches, and 32.4% children without recurrent headaches (34). The relation among the members of the nuclear family (contingency quotient of 0.429) is significantly stronger than the relation to the members of wider family (contingency quotient of 0.338) (34). The probability of a child having the migraine headache, and not the non-migraine one calculated from authors was 0.664 for a mother, 0.644 for a father, 0.411 for a father's mother, - 0.175 for a mother's mother, 0.165 for a mother's father, and – 0.102 for a father's father having similar recurrent headaches (34).

Family and twin studies show that there is a genetic component to migraine headache, but no genes predisposing to common forms of the disorder have been identified, and the actual types of genes responsible are still not fully understood (47,48).

Knežević-Pogančev and coauthors investigate headache heritability among 396 twin pairs (42.4% monozygotic and 57.6% dizygotic) aged 3 to 21 years, on north part territory of Serbia -Vojvodina

(34). Within the group of tested twin persons, 30.2% had recurrent headaches, 9.2% migraine headache and 21% other non-migraine recurrent headaches. Heritability quotient of all recurrent headaches was 0.3882. For non-migraine headaches heritability quotient of 0.2286 confirmed that the external factors influence is higher than heritability. Migraine headache heritability quotient 0.8598 clearly proved the heritability of the migraine headache. Migraine headache correlation and determination quotient of twins (monozygotic and dizygotic) shows high degree of migraine headache twin siblings dependence, and higher correlation and significance of the difference with monozygotic twins. The migraine headache of one twin is directly dependent on the migraine of the other. This mutual dependence is different for monozygotic and dizygotic twins. The analysis of such mutual influence was calculated through the correlation and determination quotient, by method of co-variant. The very high correlation quotient of the migraine headache of all twins 0.7498 the is (0.8458 of monozygotic and 0.6342 of dizygotic) and the determination quotient of the migraine headache for all the twins 56.12% (71.54% for monozygotic, and 40.22% for dizygotic twins) show that the high degree of mutual dependence between the migraine headache of twin siblings, is more important with monozygotic twins (38).

No empirical study has explicitly examined how genetic and environmental factors influence migraine headache as well as other recurrent headaches.

Migraine headache trigger factors

Various exogenous factors (triggering factors), alone or in combination with other exogenous or endogenous factors, have high tendency to provoke migraine headache in people who are prone for migraine headache. Trigger factors are exclusive occurrences, which decompensate the nervous system, provoking headache. They do not cause headaches, they just provoke them. Certain triggers do not induce headaches in everyone (49). A specific trigger may not cause head pain each time even in the apparent migraine headache sufferer. There are a lot of migraine headache triggering factors but the mechanisms by which they produce migraine headache attacks are unknown. Trigger factors are important for two main reasons: firstly, they may provide some clues to the pathogenesis of migraine headache; secondly, by avoiding them, migraine headache drug therapy may be obviated (50).

The current studies have identified over 300 different migraine headache triggers but the mechanisms by which they produce migraine headache attacks are mostly unknown (51). The prevalence and characterization of migraine headache triggers have not been rigorously studied in children and adolescents. A questionnaire study in 102 children and adolescents showed the mean number of migraine headache triggers reported per subject was 7 (52). Mean time elapsed between exposure to a trigger factor and attack onset was comprised between 0 and 3^h in 88 patients (86%). The most common individual trigger was stress (75.5% of patients); followed by lack of sleep (69.6%), warm climate (68.6%) and video games (64.7%). Stress was also the most frequently reported migraine headache trigger always associated with attacks (24.5%). In conclusion, trigger factors were frequently reported by children and adolescents with migraine headache and stress was the most frequent (52). In descending order of frequency they were cited as: sensorial stimuli (75%), sleep deprivation (49%), hunger (48%), environmental factors (47%), food (46%), menses (39%), fatigue (35%), alcohol (28%), sleep excess (27%), caffeine (22%), physical exertion (20%), head trauma (20%), trips (4%), sexual activity (3%), medications (2%), neck movements (2%), smoking (1%) and the use of a low pillow (1%) (54). Annequin D. found that migraine headache episodes in children are frequently triggered by several factors: emotional stress (school pressure, vexation, excitement, upset), hypoglycemia, lack or excess of sleep (weekend migraine), sensorial stimulation (loud noise, bright light, strong odour, warmth or cold), sympathetic stimulation (sport, physical exercise) (54). Spierings et al., reported stress/tension, not eating in time, fatigue, and lack of sleep as the most common triggers of migraine headache (55). The weather, smell, and smoke have been reported as factors that distinguished migraine headache from the tension-type headache. Nowadays, as the most common trigger factors of children migraine headache are reported: certain dietary factors, kinetosis, emotional stress, sleep deprivation, physical activity and exertion, mild hypoglycemia due to skipping meals, excessive sun exposure, high external temperature, starvation, febrile illness, different medications and various chemical substances, photo-stimulation, noise, intensive odours, etc. Only a small number of them is well studied and adequately documented in children.

Since the time of Hippocrates and Areteus of Cappadocia, there have been numerous anecdotes about foods that can trigger headaches in susceptible individuals. Schaumberg in 1969. described the "Hot dog headaches", caused by nitrates. Henderson and Raskin in 1972, and Patfield in 1995. claim alcohol as a migraine headache trigger factor. Kohlenberg in 1982. described tyramine, as a triggers for migraine headache attack. Bresolin in 1991, Barbirolli in 1992. and Montagna in 1994. described the mitochondrial relation illnesses and migraine headaches, which Boles in 1999. proved to be present among children with cyclical vomiting.

There is an amazing similarity between their observations and current knowledge of dietary triggers of migraine headaches (55). Despite a series of experimental studies demonstrating that food and odors cause headache their role remains unclear. The importance of chocolate has been doubted seriously, and scientific evidence for cheese as a precipitating factor is lacking. In spite of series of experimental studies, it is suggested that subjective sensitivity to certain foods should be examined critically, and proven trigger factors should be avoided.

General dietary restrictions have not been proven to be useful. Nowadays, as the most common trigger factors of adolescent migraine headache are reported: certain dietary factors, kinetosis, emotional stress, sleep deprivation, physical activity and exertion, mild hypoglycemia due to skipping meals, excessive sun exposure, high external temperature, starvation, febrile illness, different medications and various chemical substances, photo-stimulation, noise, intensive odours, smoke, alcohol abuse etc. Although sleep problems are a common complaint in migraine headache patients, the role of sleep habits and hygiene, as triggers of head pain, have been poorly analyzed. Only a small number of them is well studied and adequately documented in adolescents (56).

There are presented papers proving characteristic of migraine is more associated with stressful experiences than this is the case for tension-type headache. This suggests that adolescent migraine headache patients might especially benefit from behavioral interventions regarding stress (57). In our largest study of children and adolescents autors did not found the same (10).

Karl N. et al., suggested that similar trigger factors may trigger similar mechanisms and may cause common pre-headache signs and symptoms in all headache types (58). Trigger factors are important for two main reasons: firstly, they may provide some clues to the pathogenesis of migraine headache; secondly, by avoiding them, migraine headache drug therapy may be obviated (53, 59, 60).

Adolescents from the 10th and 11th grades of high schools answered questionnaires on their headaches and on potential risk factors regarding lifestyle, stress and muscle pain. Individuals reporting to have experienced headache in the preceding 6 months were asked to report what they believed to cause their headache (self-perceived triggers). 1,047 (83 %) of 1,260 adolescents reported headaches. Stress, lack of sleep and too much school work were the most frequently reported self-perceived triggers of headache; in contrast the statistical analysis identified alcohol and coffee consumption, smoking, neck pain, stress and physical inactivity as risk factors for headache. The role of stress was overestimated. The high prevalence of the other confirmed risk factors in adolescents with headache suggests potential for prevention by increasing awareness for these risk factors and appropriate interventions.

Material and methods

This research was carried out in North Serbian Province, Vojvodina, with total population of 2,031,992. Study was carried out from 1988 to 2008.

Participants were selected by multi-study random sampling procedure in 9 cities. Total of 20,917 adolescents, aged 10-18 have been included. Adolescents were selected according to their month and year of birth, and the first 3 letters of their first name – applying a multistage, stratified, clustered sampling procedure. This ensured that adolescent could not enter the study twice during the long research period. Questionnaires were given to the participants, who were drawn from 23 preschools and 42 grade schools in 9 cities in Vojvodina (Novi Sad, Subotica, Kikinda, Zrenjanin, Vršac, Bela Crkva, Melenci, Futog and Temerin).

Adolescents and/or their parents were asked to fill out a questionnaire in their places of residence. Questionnaires were distributed to children and/or their parents, selected by random sampling. The semi structured questionnaire, developed for this study by the author, and designed according to the International Headache Society criteria (IHS). It was a screening questionnaire, which was completed by children and/or their parents. It included 3 sections: (1) items about the child's socio-demographic characteristics and his/her family and school; (2) items about the child's development, and (3) items about headaches including all characteristics, signs and symptoms. The questionnaire was developed in 3 phases. First, semi structured interviews with pediatricians and researchers were organized to select relevant domains. The domains for the section about headaches were selected based on the International Classification of Headache Disorders – 2nd criteria (61). The accuracy of the questionnaire used in this survey was based on International Headache Society criteria. Using the society's classification codes, migraine headache was accepted as 1.1–1.7, migraine headache with aura was 1.2.2–1.2.6, migraine headache without aura was 1.1 and other migraine syndromes were 1.3–1.7. Recurrent headache was accepted as all headache types that appeared 1 to 3 times per month, without separating them due to specific characteristics. All types of recurrent headache (idiopathic or cryptogenic) that were not migraine headache were considered as non-migraine headaches (62, 63).

More than 150 possible items were identified. Precise, comprehensive and appropriate items were included in the first form. The possible responses were open-ended options or categorical judgments. In the second phase, the questionnaire was pretested in the semi-structured interviews

16

with a small group of adolescents who either did or did not suffer from headaches (16 families were included). This phase aimed to evaluate the questionnaire's interface and validate the content. Additionally, the sensitivity was evaluated by correlating the data from the questionnaire and the medical records of the adolescents who had headaches. This phase resulted in a revised version, which was cross-evaluated only on healthy adolescents. Fifty adolescents have completed the questionnaire twice in 3 weeks. The nonresponsive rate, response distributions, graphical response presentation (response inconsistency) and questionnaire burdens (time to complete, formatting, etc.) were analyzed. A number of items were modified or eliminated and the final form included 93 items which required 20 min to complete.

The inclusion criteria were:

- age 10–18,
- attending school,
- signed informed consent by both, parents and adolescents.

The exclusion criterion was:

- prior diagnosis of a disease that has a headache as a symptom.

The World Health Organization (WHO) defines adolescence as the period of life with psychological and social transition between childhood and adulthood, i.e. from the age of 10 to the age of 19. We included ages from 10 to 18 according to the Health Care rules in Serbia. The mean age of the participants was 15 years and 2.5 months (range 10–18 years, SD 3.02).

The study was approved by Ethical Committees of the Institute and the University of Novi Sad. All patients and their parents have signed the informed consent before entering the study.

The study was conducted in 3 phases.

- first phase of the study was completing a questionnaire to narrow down the number of patients to those who had at least two headaches per month over the past year.
- second phase was a face-to-face interview, as well as physical and neurological examination. After diagnosing migraine headache, adolescents with migraine headache were asked to keep a headache diary over the period of 6 months. In addition, they were asked to strictly avoid potential triggers, and continue keeping the headache dairy.
- third phase was re-interviewing them one year after they started the headache and medication diary.

Due to the possible duplicate interviews (1.5%) and due to the incomplete questionnaires - 5.5% of findings have been biased. Questionnaires completely answered by adolescents who had RH were analyzed separately. Comparing characteristics of individual headaches in adolescents with migraine headaches and non-migraine headaches, specific age dependent features of migraine headaches were established.

The demographics, clinical and social characteristics were described by age and sex according to headache presence and type. The Hi2 test, Levin test and ANOVA were used as statistical methods. A significance level of 5% was used (p<0.05). All statistical analyses were performed with SPSS 15.0 (SPSS Inc., Chicago, Ill., USA).

Results

Adolescents filled out the questionnaire (20,917), 4,376 (20.9 %) of them reported recurrent headaches, and 2,008 (9.4%) of them reported migraine headache (1020 girls and 988 boys). Out of 20,917 adolescents, 4,376 (20.9%) reported recurrent non-migraine headache, and 2008 (9.4%) reported migraine headache.

Migraine headache with aura was diagnosed in 514 (25.6%) adolescents, migraine headache without aura in 1349 (67.2%) and other migraine syndromes in 145 (7.2%) adolescents. Migraine headache was reported for the first time in children aged 5 years 2.4 months, migraine headache with aura in children aged 4 years 11.4 months, migraine headache without aura in children aged 5years 7.2 months, and other migraine headaches syndromes in children aged 3 years 7.2 months (Table 1. Headache according to age with first attack)

Table 1. Headache - age at first attack

Migraine headache type	f	Age on first attack	Standard deviation	Standard error of the arithmetical mean
-with aura	514	4 y 11.4 m	1.05	0.04
-without aura	1349	5 y 7.2 m	1.37	0.04
-other migraine syndromes	145	3 y 7.2 m	0.58	0.05
Migraine headache	2008	5y 1.8m	1.47	0.03

ANOVA F 79.215, DF 7, Sig 0.0001

Pulsating pain is most frequent in adolescents migraine headaches (76.3%), whereas undefined (30.1%), pressure (29.8%) and squeezing pain (24.6%) are more frequent in non-migraine headaches.

Pulsating head pain is the most frequent in adolescents with migraine headache aged over 12 years, while squeezing is the most frequent head pain in adolescents with non migraine headache aged 11 years 3 months, and pressing is the most frequent in adolescent aged 11 years 1,7 months. The younger the child, the more likely is that the pain will be described as undefined (Grafic 1. Head pain type)

Grafic 1. Head pain type

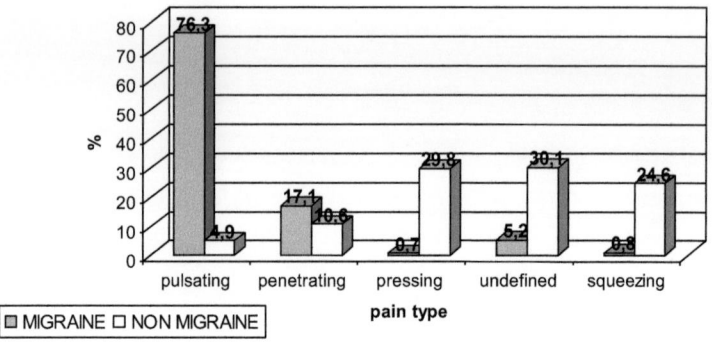

Adolescents with migraine headaches older than 10 years assessed their pain severity using a Pain Assessment Scale of 0 – 5 with 3.68, at age 13 years 5.7months (range 10-18years) (Table 2. Pain intensity assessment and the age of examinees).

Table 2. Pain intensity assessment and the age of examinees

Pain intensity assessment // Age	f	Arithmetical mean	Standard deviation	Pearson's coefficient of correlation	Statistical significance of correlation coefficient
Age of examinees		13 y 5.7m	3.44		
Pain intensity assessment	2008	3.68	0.84	0.41	0.01

Migraine head pain is mostly unilateral (79.4% of all) at age 14years 5 month. Migraine headache was mostly unilateral followed by bilateral pain at age 11years 2.2 months (11.5% of all), and mostly bilateral at age 10years 7 months in 7.7% of all adolescent migraine headaches (Table 3. Headache pain location regarding to age).

Tabela 3. **Headache pain location regarding to age**

Headaches	Migraine headaches	
Pain location//Age	%	Arith. mean
Unilateral	79.4	14y 5.0m
Bilateral	7.7	10y 7.0m
Various	1.4	10y 5.m
Unilateral and then bilateral	11.5	11y 2.2 m

ANOVA: F 227.352, DF 5, Sig 0.0001

Migraine headache appears usually several times per year after 13th birthday, but during earlier years of life it appears weekly, even daily (Table 4. Frequency and type of headache, age on examinees).

Table 4. **Frequency and type of headache, age on examinees**

Headaches	Migraine	
Age	%	arith. means
Several a month	6.1	10y 2.8m
Several a year	78.1	13y 1.5m
Variable	15.8	11y 0.2m

ANOVA   F 22.542, DF 7, Sig 0.0001 – Headaches, generally
ANOVA   F 13.071, DF 7, Sig 0.0001 – Non-migraine

Nausea, vomiting impulse and vomiting are much more frequent in younger adolescents. Only 8.3% of adolescent with migraine headaches of average age 13 years and 4.8 months do not have nausea, vomiting instinct and vomiting (Table 5. Migraine headache associated nausea and vomiting in regard to the age).

Table 5. **Migraine headache associated nausea and vomiting in regard to the age**

Headaches	Nausea Vomiting instinct and Vomiting	%	Arithmetical mean	Standard deviation	Standard error of the arithmetical mean	Statistical significance of differences
Migraine headaches	No	8.3	13y 4.8m	2.31	0.25	
	Yes	91.7	13y 2m	3.00	0.07	0.001
	TOTAL	100	11y 1.0m	3.04	0.07	

Free sample test : F 33.315, t– 9.6222, DF 6595, Sig 0.0001

There was not found out age dependency for other accompanying migraine headache symptoms (photophobia, phonohobia, vertigo, skin pallor, dark circles under the eyes, sweating, irregular breathing, precordial pain and other vegetative symptoms, noticeable behavior changes), as well as in coping with migraine reporting in observed children.

Among the adolescents with migraine headache in our group we do not find any confirmation of "migraine personality". Parents of adolescents with the migraine headache described them as ambitious and over-sensitive, but more frequently as non-striking (Table 6. Presence and type of headache according to pattern of behavior).

Table 6 - Presence and type of headache according to pattern of behavior

Child's nature	Withdrawn introvert	Over-sensitive	Too conscientious	Restless	Ambitious	Not striking
Headaches	%	%	%	%	%	%
Without headaches	13.4	7.1	0.4	26.6	2.3	50.2
Migraine headaches	10.5	23.6	0.2	13.3	24.8	**27.6**
Other headaches	11.6	8.8	0.3	23.7	8.6	47.0
TOTAL	12.8	8.8	0.3	24.9	5.4	47.6

Pearson Chi Square: V 2758.93023, DF 10, Sig 0.000001

Adolescents with migraine headaches were significantly less frequently described as non-striking (27.6%), in comparison to adolescents without headaches (50.2%) and adolescents with non-migraine headaches (47.0%), which certainly represents not clear enough a particularity at this moment, the recognition of which is the basal aim of this research.

Parents most frequently describe their children (adolescents) suffering from migraine headache with aura as being non-striking, over-sensitive and ambitious, and less often as withdrawn and restless. Adolescents suffering from migraine headache without aura, parents describe as ambitious, non-striking, over-sensitive, restless, withdrawn and too conscientious. The characteristics of the pattern of behavior of adolescents with migraine headache equivalents, parents define as restless, over-sensitive, withdrawn and non-striking. It has been found that migraine headache without aura is significantly more present among all the adolescents whose pattern of behavior has been described as being borderline or extreme. All this speaks in favor of the assumption that emotional and psychological changes have stronger influence on demonstration of the migraine headache without aura, and on its less clear genetic determination in comparison to migraine headache with aura (Table 7. Migraine headache according to pattern of behavior).

Table 7 – Migraine headache according to pattern of behavior

Pattern of behavior	Withdrawn introvert	Over-sensitive	Too conscientious	Restless	Ambitious	Not striking
Migraine headache	%	%	%	%	%	%
With aura	7.7	31.1	-	5.1	22.3	33.8
Without aura	10.0	20.3	0.3	14.1	28.4	26.8
Others	24.7	28.0	-	34.0	-	13.3
TOTAL	**10.5**	**23.6**	**0.2**	**13.3**	**24.8**	**27.6**

Pearson Chi Square: V 195.79153, DF 10, Sig 0.000001

Migraine headache is significantly more present among the second-born children in the family 1,070 (53.3%) than among the first-born ones 938 (46.7%) or other children 20 (1%).

Migraine headache is more frequent (10.4%) among adolescents coming from incomplete families, with bad family atmosphere (9.1%); the most frequent is migraine headache without aura which appears in 57.1%. Adolescents with migraine headaches significantly more often come from families where mother is the dominant figure (61.2%); it is the outcome of over-protectiveness on mother`s behalf, or continual stress due to inadequate projections of a mother onto a child. There are no significant statistical differences in presence of types of migraine headache when related to the dominance of a particular family figure (mother, father, other).

Migraine headache is more present among adolescents living in families of "poor material status ". 36.1% of registered adolescents come from these families, 55.6% of them come from families of "middle material status", and only 8.1% of them from families of "good material status". Among the migraine headaches important is the predominance of migraine without aura in the families of poor material status (Pearson Chi Square: V 08.93736; DF3; Sig 0.000001) (Table 8. Migraine headache according to a material status of the family).

Table 8. Migraine headache according to a material status of the family

Material status of the family	Poor		Middle		Good	
Migraine headache	f	%	f	%	f	%
With aura	122	23.0	382	**72.1**	26	4.9
Without aura	572	**41.0**	697	50.0	125	9.0
Other migraine	54	36.0	78	52.0	18	12.0
TOTAL	748	36.1	1157	55.8	169	8.1

Pearson Chi Square: V 79.22895, DF 4, Sig 0.000001

Migraine headaches were more present among adolescents not attending the local school (in a place where they live), (16.42%:11.89%), which can be explained by a number of provoking factors (getting up early in the morning, not enough sleep, not cooked meals at school, driving by bus, etc.).

The length of breast-feeding period was analyzed on 20,008 adolescents, for whom the data have been available, by a method of variants, multiple level tests and Scheffe test with significance level less than 0.0001. Adolescents suffering from migraine headache without aura were breast-fed for a significantly shorter time than adolescents suffering from other migraine headaches, especially than the adolescents suffering from migraine headache with aura. Adolescents with migraine headache without aura were breast-fed for 3.5 months and 27 days on average; adolescents with other migraine headaches were breast-fed for 4 months and 5.1 days, and children with migraine headache with aura for 5 months and 18.9 days. The obtained result reveals a completely new, ultra-early disposition factor of the migraine headache- the "length of breast-feeding period", and it requires further metabolic investigation of the influence of breast-feeding on the migraine syndrome (Table 9. Headache type according to the length of breast-feeding period).

Negative Pearson`s correlation quotient clearly shows the reciprocal influence of the length of breast-feeding period on the appearance of migraine headache, i.e. the earlier demonstration of the migraine headache among adolescents who were breast-fed for a shorter time. The length of breast-feeding period not only directly influences the appearance of the migraine headache in general, but the age when it appears as well. Migraine headache appears among younger groups of adolescents breast-fed for a shorter period of time.

Table 9. Headache type according to the length of breast-feeding period

Types of headaches	Breast-feeding // age when the headache appeared	f	Arithmetic means	Standard deviation	Pearson`s correlation quotient	Statistical significance of the correlation quotient
SUM TOTAL	Breast-feeding	603	4.90	3.04	0.15	0.01
	age when the headache appeared		5.76	1.69		
Other	Breast-feeding	4007	5.14	3.02	0.18	0.01
	age when the headache appeared		6.23	1.68		
Migraine headache	Breast-feeding	2012	4.36	2.45	**-0.07**	0.01
	age when the headache appeared		5.20	1.47		
With aura	Breast-feeding	527	5.63	2.28	**-0.01**	0.01
	age when the headache appeared		4.83	1.05		
Without aura	Breast-feeding	1373	3.90	2.28	**-0.01**	0.01
	age when the headache appeared		5.59	1.37		
Other migraine	Breast-feeding	127	4.17	2.92	0.11	0.01
	age when the headache appeared		2.56	0.58		

Adolescents with migraine headaches were given the ready-made industrial food (ANOVA: F141.0590, DF2, Sig 0.00001) earlier, which is in an inverse proportion to the length of breast-feeding period. The analysis of the variant and multiple levels test (Scheffe) confirm the statistically very important difference in age when the ready-made industrial food was introduced into eating (ANOVA: F95.2834, DF2, Sig 0.00001). Negative Pearson`s correlation quotient and its statistical importance of 0.01, confirm that the early introduction of industrially made food into child`s eating, leads to earlier demonstration of the migraine.

By analyzing the psychomotor development (age at which a child can sit, stand, walk, vocalize, talk, control sphincters by day and/or night on its own...), as well as by comparing the adolescents with the migraine headache, adolescents without headaches and those with non-migraine headaches, and by a method of variant, the following result was obtained: the differences were statistically minimal and meaningless, on the level of a day, with no practical value, and require no further interpretation and processing.

7881 adolescents were included into the investigation of the influence of the child`s early joining in the nursery school on a whole-day stay basis; 6412 of them (81.36%) without headaches, 305 of them (3.87%) with migraine headaches, and 1164 (14.77%) of them with non-migraine headaches. Migraine headache was more often found (39.4%) among those adolescents who were younger when joined to a whole-day stay basis in nursery schools (ANOVA: F278.99704, DF1, and Sig 0.05). Important is the difference among the length of a stay in a group for the children without headaches (1 year, 8 months and 24 days), for the children with non-migraine headaches (2 years and 27 days), and the children with migraine headaches (3 years, 1 month and 12 days) (Table 10- Appearance and type of headache according to joining a group).

Table 10 – Appearance and type of headache according to joining a group

Stay at a nursery school (age) // Headaches	f	Arithmetic means	Standard deviation	Standard error of arithmetic means
Without headache	6412	**1.74**	1.00	0.01
Migraine headaches	305	**3.12**	1.52	0.09
Other headaches	1164	**2.08**	1.25	1.04
Migraine headache with aura	20	**3.00**	1.45	0.32
Migraine headache without aura	135	**3.57**	1.39	0.12
Other migraine headaches	150	**2.73**	1.54	0.13
TOTAL	305	**3.12**	1.52	0.09

ANOVA: F 278.9704, DF 1, Sig 0.05
ANOVA: F 11.7309, DF 2, Sig 0.05

Table 11 – Specific disposition factors according to a type of headache

Specific disposition factors	Recurrent abdominal pain		Episodic vertigo		Somnabulism		Paroxysmal torticollis	
Headaches	f	%	f	%	f	%	f	%
Migraine headaches	434	24.6	135	43	652	31.4	139	6.5
Other headaches	148	4.4	19	**2.6**	544	**12.0**	19	0.4
SUM TOTAL	582	11.4	184	0.8	1886	7.8	183	0.8

Recurrent abdominal pain: Pearson Chi Square: V 67.163 , DF 1, Sig 0.0001
Episodic vertigo: Pearson Chi Square: V 406.051, DF 1, Sig 0.0001
Somnambulism: Pearson Chi Square: V 2069.74259, DF 2, Sig 0.000001
Paroxysmal Torticollis: Pearson Chi Square: V 986.90245, DF 2, Sig 0.000001

Adolescents with migraine headache scoped within the investigated sample, have the particularities which can be considered as being disposition factors of the migraine headache among adolescents (Table 11. Specific disposition factors according to a type of headache).

Very high specific disposition factors according to a type of headache are:

- recurrent abdominal pain in anamnesis, in 24.6% (31.2% of adolescents having migraine headache with aura and 21.9% of adolescents having the migraine headache without aura),
- episodic vertigo of unclear etiology which cannot be considered as being benign paroxysmal vertigo in anamnesis (43% of adolescents with migraine headache and 2.6% adolescents with non-migraine headaches),
- somnambulism among 31.4% of adolescents with migraine headaches, 12.0% with non-migraine ones, and 4% without headaches,
- Primary intrauterine torticollis among 6.5% of adolescents with migraine headaches.

Kinetosis is highly present among the adolescents with the migraine syndrome. Only 0.3% of adolescent who have no record of kinetosis, have the migraine headache, while the non-migraine headache appears among them in 13.2%. Among adolescents suffering kinetosis, migraine headache appears in 21.0% while non-migraine one appears in 21.6%. Adolescents with migraine headaches had kinetosis in 92.8% (65% with migraine with aura; 92.7% with migraine without aura; 96.7% with migraine equivalents), while adolescents with non-migraine headaches had kinetosis in 25.1% and adolescents without headaches in 12.0% .

Different, though often unclear recurrent vegetative symptomatology (vertigo, dizziness, collapses, nausea, change of skin color, perspiration etc.) in a personal anamnesis, is statistically highly significantly present among the adolescents with migraine headache (43.0%), when compared to the adolescents with headaches of non-migraine headache etiology.

In a group of left-handed adolescents the migraine headache is present among 2.3% of them, non-migraine headaches among 33.1% of them, while there is no record of recurrent headaches. In a group of right-handed adolescents, the migraine headache is present among 7.8% of adolescents and non-migraine headache among 18.2% of them.

In the group of adolescents with insufficient brain hemisphere dominance even 18.6% had migraine headache, 14.9% of them had non-migraine headaches, while 66.4% of them had not record recurrent headaches. Among adolescents having the migraine headache 1.8% were left-handed, 73.8% were right-handed, and even 24.4% of them were adolescents with insufficient brain hemisphere dominance. 10.2% of the total number of the entire migraine headache with aura, 27.3% of the entire migraine headache without aura, and 47.3% of all the other migraine headaches, appear in the case of insufficient coincidence of gestural and applicable lateralization. Lesser

26

presence of both left-handed and right-handed adolescents with a significant rise in presence of insufficient brain hemisphere dominance within the group of adolescents with the migraine headache, clearly shows the relation between the brain hemisphere dominance and migraine headache (Table 12. Headache type according to gestural : applicable lateralization).

Table 12- Types of headaches according to gestural : applicable lateralization

Gestural lateralization	Left-handed		Bi manuel		Right-handed	
Headaches	f	%	f	%	f	%
Without headache	1062	6.1	1805	10.4	14570	83.6
Migraine headaches	38	1.8	506	24.4	1530	73.8
Other headaches	544	12.0	406	9.0	3575	79.0
Migraine with aura	5	0.9	54	10.2	471	88.9
Migraine without aura	22	1.6	381	27.3	991	71.1
Migraine equivalents	11	7.3	71	47.3	68	45.3
SUM TOTAL	1644	6.8	2717	11.3	19675	81.9

Pearson Chi Square: V 645.550, DF 4, Sig 0.000001
Pearson Chi Square: V 645.550, DF 4, Sig 0.0001
Left-handed – gestural lateralization with applicable left-handed 7:3 to 10:0 left;

Right-handed – gestural lateralization with applicable right-handed 7:3 to 10:0 right;

BI – gestural lateralization, 6:4 or less, in relation to the side of applicable lateralization.

Migraine headache appeared earlier with and more frequently among the adolescents with insufficient coincidence of gestural and applicable lateralization. With left-handed adolescents migraine headache was more often demonstrated at a medium age of 6 years and 7.2 months, with right-handed children at a medium age of 6 years and 10.3 months. In adolescents with insufficient coincidence of gestural and applicable lateralization, migraine headache most frequently appeared at a medium age of 5 years and 6.4 months.

Influence of the insufficient brain hemisphere dominance of insufficient coincidence of gestural and applicable lateralization with its importance of p<0,000001, allows its presence among the disposition factors of the migraine headache. Having in mind that it is objective, able to undergo test evaluation and assessment, as well as early recognizable, it has an enormous practical importance. In order to separate persons with a high risk of the migraine headache, it is necessary to test the applicable and gestural lateralization of all children.

If the inherited substrate of the migraine headache is a metabolic disorder, or disorders that lead to instability and excessive reaction of the neural-vasomotor system, then there must be other manifestation of this state as well, with clear clinical display as can be seen with the migraine headache: cyclical vomiting and periodical syndromes. Thus, these disorders can be considered to be a basal disposition for kinetosis, somnambulism, orthostatic circulatory insufficiency and allergy - the same as the migraine headache.

Clearly identified and statistically significant headache triggers were established in 10.4% of adolescents with non-migraine headaches and in 3.9% of adolescents with migraine headaches. Clear triggers as direct causes of migraine headache attacks were most significant for occurrence of migraine headache without aura (Table 13. Direct headache triggering factors).

Table 13. Direct headache triggering factors

Presence of triggering factors	No		Yes	
Recurrent headaches	f	%	f	%
Non-migraine headaches	3921	89.6	455	10.4
Migraine headaches	1930	96.1	78	3.9
Migraine with aura	501	97.9	13	2.1
Migraine without aura	1302	96.8	47	3.2
Other migraine headaches	120	83.3	25	16.7

Pearson Chi Square: V 79.02093, DF 1, Sig 0.000001
Pearson Chi square: V 71.52128, DF 2, Sig 0.00001

Adolescents with non-migraine headaches are more susceptible to weather changes than adolescents with migraine headaches (Sig 0.000001). Individuals suffering from migraine headache without aura are most susceptible to weather conditions, in regard to those suffering from other migraine headache (Sig 0.001). Only 16.3% of adolescents with migraine headache with aura, and 77.95% of adolescents with migraine headache without aura identified weather changes as a direct migraine headache trigger factor. This clearly confirms significantly higher effects of weather conditions on occurrence of non-migraine headache in regard to migraine headaches in adolescents (Sig 0.000001) (Table 14. Weather conditions (meteoropathy) as a headache trigger factor).

Table 14. Weather conditions (meteoropathy) as a headache triggering factor

Weather conditions (Meteoropathy)	No		Yes	
Recurrent headaches	f	%	f	%
Non-migraine headaches	2768	61.2	1608	38.8
Migraine headaches	1580	78.7	428	21.3
Migraine with aura	430	83.7	84	16.3
Migraine without aura	298	22.1	851	77.9
Other migraine headaches	109	75.3	36	24.7

Pearson Chi Square: V 10.7188, DF 1, Sig 0.001
Pearson Chi Square: V 161.40034, DF 1, Sig 0.000001

In the group of girls without premenstrual syndrome, presence of migraine headache with aura (27.3%) and migraine headache without aura (72.7%) corresponds to the rate in the general population. In the group of girls with migraine headache associated premenstrual syndrome, 45.3%

had migraine headache with aura and 54.7% had migraine headache without aura. The effects of hormonal factors on migraine headache generally speaking, and on migraine headache with aura, are significantly higher than on non-migraine recurrent headaches (Sig 0.0002). 46.3% of girls presented with migraine headache with aura and premenstrual syndrome. In the group of girls with migraine headache without aura, 71.9% did not have premenstrual syndrome, and 28.1% presented with premenstrual syndrome.

In the group of adolescents indicating overexertion (fatigue) as a trigger factor, 32.8% of all headaches are migraine headaches, and 67.2% are non-migraine headaches, which corresponds with relations between migraine headache (31.4%) and non-migraine headaches (68.6%) in all examined adolescents. Overexertion cannot be considered as a migraine headache trigger in adolescents, although it is often claimed to be a migraine headache trigger in adults.

Usually physical activity tends to trigger non-migraine headaches (84.1%) more often than migraine headaches (74.5%) (Sig 0.0001). Among migraine headaches, usually physical activity is a more frequent trigger of migraines headaches without aura (Sig 0.0001) (Table 15. Effects of usually physical activity on headache occurrence).

Table 15. Effects of usually physical activity on headache occurrence

Effects of physical activity	No		Yes	
Headaches	f	%	f	%
Non-migraine headaches	696	15.9	3680	84.1
Migraine headaches	512	25.5	1496	74.5
Migraine with aura	206	40.2	308	59.8
Migraine without aura	266	19.6	0193	80.4
Migraine equivalents 145	30	20,7	115	79,3

Pearson Chi Square: V 69510, DF 1, Sig 0.0001
Pearson Chi Square: V 81.194, DF 1, Sig 0.0001

In the group of adolescents with migraine headache who indicated overexertion as a trigger factor of migraine headache attacks, 25.7% have migraine headache with aura, and 67.7% have migraine headache without aura, whereas 6.6% have other migraine headaches. This corresponds with findings related with migraine headache in the examined population. However, physical exertion cannot be attributed importance in triggering certain migraine headaches. There is no significant difference in the group of adolescents with recurrent headaches (92.3%), non-migraine headaches (93.1%) and migraine headaches (99.2%) (Table 16. Physical exertion as a headache triggering factor).

Table 16. Physical exertion as a headache triggering factor

Effects of physical exertion	No		Yes	
Recurrent headaches	f	%	f	%
Non-migraine headaches	302	6.9	4074	93.1
Migraine headaches	16	0.8	1992	99.2
Migraine with aura	1	0.2	513	99.8
Migraine without aura	1	0.1	1348	99.9
Other migraine headaches	14	10.0	131	90.0

Pearson Chi Square: V 11.851, DF 1, Sig 0.0001
Pearson Chi Square: V 167.692, DF 2, Sig 0.0001

Food deprivation (short-term insufficient food intake) significantly affects occurrence of non-migraine headache in regard to migraine headaches (Sig 0.0001) (Table 17.Effects of food deprivation on migraine headache occurrence).

Table 17. Effects of food deprivation on migraine headache occurrence

Effects of food deprivation	No		Yes	
Recurrent headaches	f	%	f	%
Non-migraine headaches	3286	75.1	1090	24.9
Migraine headaches	1600	79.7	408	20.3
Migraine with aura	424	82.5	90	17.5
Migraine without aura	1080	80.1	269	19.9
Other migraine syndromes	97	66.7	48	33.3

Pearson Chi Square: V 16.901, DF 1 Sig 0.0001
Likelihood Ratio: V 16.610, DF 2, Sig 0.0001

In the group of adolescents in whom food deprivation is not a trigger of migraine headache attacks, 32.4% suffer from migraine headaches and 67.3% suffer from non-migraine headaches. Among adolescents who indicate food deprivation as a migraine headache trigger, 27.2% have migraine headache and 72.8% have non-migraine headaches. Food deprivation as a triggering factor of migraines headache is much more frequent in adolescents with non-migraine headache than in adolescents with migraine headaches (24.9%:20.3%). (Table 17. Effects of food deprivation on migraine headache occurrence).

Migraine headaches are much more frequent (89.8%) than non-migraine headaches (58.4%) in adolescents with motion sickness (kinetosis) as a direct headache trigger (Sig 0.0001) (Table 18. Effects of kinetosis (motion sickness) on migraine headache occurrence).

Table 18. Effects of kinetosis on migraine headache occurrence

Effects of motion sickness	No		Yes	
Recurrent headaches	f	%	f	%
Non-migraine headaches	1820	41.6	2556	**58.4**
Migraine headaches	205	10.2	1803	**89.8**
Migraine with aura	69	13.4	445	86.6
Migraine without aura	101	7.5	1248	92.5
Other migraine headaches	34	23.3	111	76.7

Fisher Exact Test: V 735.350, DF 1, Sig 0.0001
Fisher Exact Test and Likelihood Ratio: V 735.350, DF 1, Sig 0.0001

In the group of adolescents with migraine headaches who indicated kinetosis as a triggering factor of migraine headache attacks, 24.6% have migraine headache with aura, and 69.2% have migraine headache without aura, and 6.2% have other migraine headaches. Kinetosis or travel sickness equally triggers all types of migraine headache (Sig 0.0001) (Table 18. Effects of kinetosis on migraine headache occurrence).

Tobacco smoke triggers migraine headaches (51.8%) much more often than non-migraine headaches (23.2%) (Sig 0.0001). Smoking is a trigger of both migraine headache (39.6%) and non-migraine (27.0%) headaches. However, smoking is a much stronger trigger of migraine headaches than of non-migraine headaches (Sig 0.0001). There is no evidence for the level of probability (p>0.03) that smoking affects interrelation of migraine headaches (Table 19. Effects of tobacco smoke on migraine headache occurrence).

Table 19. Effects of tobacco smoke on migraine headache occurrence

Effects of tobacco smoke	No		Yes	
Reccurent headaches	f	%	f	%
Non-migraine headaches	3338	76.8	1038	**23.2**
Migraine headaches	968	48.2	1040	**51.8**
Migraine with aura	220	42.8	294	57.2
Migraine without aura	635	47.1	714	52.9
Other migraine headaches	111	76.7	34	23.3

Linear-by-Linear Association, Fisher Exact Test: V 532.965, DF 1, Sig 0.0001
Pearson Chi Square: V 55.445, DF 2, Sig 0.0001

Alcohol consumption can trigger migraine headaches (44.8%) more frequently than non-migraine headaches (21.2%) (Sig 0.0001). This effect is more expressed in migraine headache with aura (60.9%) than in migraine headache without aura (36.9%). This should be taken with reserve due to the age of examinees (Sig 0.002) (Table 20. Effects of alcohol consumption on migraine headache occurrence).

Table 20. Effects of alcohol consumption on migraine headache occurrence

Effects of alcohol consumption	No		Yes	
Recurrent headaches	f	%	f	%
Non-migraine headaches	3448	78.8	828	**21.2**
Migraine headaches	1108	55.2	900	**44.8**
Migraine with aura	201	39.1	313	**60.9**
Migraine without aura	851	63.1	498	**36.9**
Other migraine headaches	107	73.8	38	**26.2**

Continuity Correlation: V 42882, DF 1, Sig 0.0001
Linear–by–Linear Association: V 9948, DF 1, Asymp Sig 0.002

Emotional factors and personality structure are of prime significance for adolescents with migraine headache. Psychological stress is often reported as a trigger factor of migraine headache, and the "school" is blamed. There are no significant differences in effects of acute stress on occurrence of migraine headache and non-migraine headaches (31.2%:68.8%) and on occurrence of certain migraine headaches. Chronic stress is reported as a direct trigger of migraine headache attacks in 26.5% of adolescents with migraine headache with aura, 70.2% of adolescents with migraine headache without aura and in 3.3% of adolescents with other migraine headaches. Chronic stress is known to be a major trigger factor of migraine headache without aura (Sig 0.0001). Chronic stress is indicated as a migraine headache trigger in 88.3% of adolescents with migraine headache with aura, 89.1% of adolescents with migraine headache without aura and in 39.3% of adolescents with other migraine headaches (Sig 0.0001). In the group of adolescents reporting chronic stress as a trigger factor of migraine headache attacks, 26.5% have migraine headache with aura, 70.2% have migraine headache without aura, and 3.3% have other migraine headaches. These findings confirm that in the examined sample chronic stress has the greatest effect on occurrence of migraine headache without aura (Table 21. Effects of chronic stress on migraine attacks).

Table 21. Effects of chronic stress on migraine attacks

Effects of chronic stress	No		Yes	
Migraine syndromes	f	%	f	%
Migraine with aura	158	11.7	1191	88.3
Migraine without aura	56	10.9	458	89.1
Other migraine headaches	88	60.7	57	39.3

Linear-by-Linear Association: V 94063. DF 2, Sig 0.0001

Oversleeping cannot be considered a trigger factor of headaches generally speaking, and it is not a trigger of migraine headache either (Table 22. Effects of oversleeping on migraine headache occurrence).

Table 22. Effects of oversleeping on migraine headache occurrence

Effects of oversleeping	No		Yes	
Recurrent headaches	f	%	f	%
Non-migraine headaches	4284	97.9	092	**2.1**
Migraine headaches	1994	99.3	14	**0.7**
Migraine with aura	510	99.4	4	**0.6**
Migraine without aura	1344	99.6	5	**0.4**
Other migraine headaches	140	96.7	5	**3.3**

Linear-by-Linear Association: V 18.553, DF 1, Sig 0.0001
Pearson Chi Square: V 17.148, DF 1, Sig 0.0001

Lack of sleep and a bad night's sleep, as direct triggers of migraine headache, are equally reported by adolescents with migraine headaches (98.6%) and by adolescents with non-migraine headaches (94.4%). Lack of sleep can trigger migraine headache attacks in all migraine headaches in adolescents (99.6% in migraine headache with aura, 99.3% in migraine headache without aura and 88.0% in migraine headaches) without clear difference in regard to effects on other migraine headaches (Table 23. Effects of lack of sleep on migraine headache occurrence).

Table 23. Effects of lack of sleep on headache occurrence

Lack of sleep	No		Yes	
Recurrent headaches	f	%	f	%
Non-migraine headaches	245	5.6	4131	**94.4**
Migraine headaches	28	1.4	1980	**98.6**
Migraine with aura	2	0.4	512	**99.6**
Migraine without aura	9	0.7	1340	**99.3**
Other migraine headaches	17	12.0	128	**88.0**

Pearson Chi Square: V 59610, DF 1, Sig 0.0001
Pearson Chi Square: V 126.641, DF 2, Sig 0.0001

Food triggers can play a huge role in non migraine headaches and migraine headaches. Even 89.1% of adolescents with migraine headaches indicated foods as triggers of migraine headache attacks, as well as 11.9% of adolescents with non-migraine headaches (Table 24. Effects of certain foods on occurrence of migraine headache attacks).

Table 24. Effects of certain foods on occurrence of migraine headache attacks

Effects of foods	No		Yes	
Recurrent headaches	f	%	7	%
Non-migraine headaches	4209	96.2	67	3.8
Migraine headaches	1297	64.6	711	35.4
Migraine with aura	371	72.3	143	27.7
Migraine without aura	834	61.8	515	38.2
Other migraine headaches	90	62.7	55	37.3

Linear-by-Linear Association: V 1203.032, DF 1, Sig 0.0001,
Linear-by-Linear Association: V 13648, DF 1, Sig 0.0001

The most common dietary headache triggers in adolescents were: cow's milk (32.43%), eggs (32.430, chocolate (29.73%), oranges (28.38%), crispy 28.38%), benzoic acid (18.92%), cheese (17.57%), tomatoes (16.22%), oregano (16.22%), fish (12.16%), pork (10.81%).

Certain odors can trigger headaches and they are 10 times more frequent in adolescents with migraine headaches than in adolescents with non-migraine headaches. In examined adolescents who reported odors as direct migraine triggers, 82.9% have migraine and 17.1% have non-migraine headaches. In adolescents who indicated odours (gasoline, sweat, other people's odors, intensive deodorants and so on) as direct trigger factors of migraine headache attacks, 18.8% have migraine headache with aura, 73.5% have migraine headache without aura and 7.7% have other migraine headaches. Certain odors have the greatest effect on occurrence of migraine headaches without aura (Table 25. Effects of odours on migraine headache occurrence).

Table 25. Effects of odors on headache occurrence

Effects of odors	No		Yes	
Recurrent headaches	f	%	f	%
Non-migraine headaches	4311	95.3	213	4.7
Migraine headaches	1040	50.2	1033	49.8
Migraine with aura	336	63.4	194	36.6
Migraine without aura	634	45.5	759	54.5
Other migraine headaches	70	46.7	80	53.3

Linear-by–Linear Association: V 1889.054, DF 1, Sig 0.0001
Likelihood Ratio: V 50.389, DF 2, Sig 0.0001

The age of adolescents is of importance when identifying foods as direct triggers of migraine headaches. Some foods are indicated as direct triggers of migraine headaches attacks by 735 adolecents, mean age 11 years and 8.9 months, whereas 1.339 adolescents, mean age 10 years and 9 months, did not indicate food as a direct trigger of migraine headache attacks. 1033 adolescent aged 11 years reported various odors as trigger factors of migraine headache attacks. This is in favor of slight, but still existing, higher susceptibility of younger children and adolescents to odours as trigger factors of migraine attacks, and vice versa in regard to foods.

Psychological stress was much more frequently reported as a direct trigger of headaches by children with non-migraine headaches (86.9%) than by adolescents with migraine headaches (13.1%) (Sig 0.0001) (Table 26. Effects of psychological stress on migraine headache occurrence).

Table 26. Effects of psychological stress on migraine headache occurrence

Effects of psychological stress	No		Yes	
Recurrent headaches	f	%	f	%
Non-migraine headaches	748	17.1	3628	82.9
Migraine headaches	1454	72.4	554	27.6
Migraine with aura	363	70.6	151	29.4
Migraine without aura	1016	75.3	333	24.7
Other migraine headaches	86	56.0	59	44.0

Likelihood Ratio: V 1935.861, DF 1, Sig 0.0001
Likelihood Ratio: V 25289, DF 2, Sig 0.0001

In the total sample of investigated adolescents with migraine headaches, 25.6% have migraine headaches with aura, 67.2% have migraine headaches without aura and 7.2% have other migraine headaches. In the group of adolescents who indicated psychological stress as a trigger factor of migraine headache attacks, 27.6% have migraine headache with aura, 60.8% have migraine headache without aura, and 11.7% have other migraine headaches . Psychological stress cannot be considered and discussed as a trigger factor of migraine headaches.

The current literature indicates that there are over 300 different trigger factors of migraine headache attacks. Numerous "other" triggering factors, which significantly interfere with activities of daily living, provoke migraine attacks a great deal in adolescents with migraine headache (81.6%) in regard to adolescent with non-migraine headaches (14.2%). "Other" factors are direct triggers in adolescents with migraine headache with aura (81.9%), in adolescents with migraine headache without aura (89.0%) and in adolescents with other migraine headaches (11.3%).

Table 27. Effects of other triggering factors on migraine headache occurrence

Other triggering factors	No		Yes	
Headaches	f	%	f	%
Non-migraine headaches	3741	85.8	635	**14.2**
Migraine headaches	369	18.4	1639	**81.6**
Migraine with aura	93	18.1	421	81.9
Migraine without aura	148	11.0	1201	89.0
Other migraine headaches	129	88.7	16	11.3

Pearson Chi Square: 2827.431, DF 1, Sig 0.0001
Pearson Chi Square: V 544049, DF 2, Sig 0.0001

On the whole, "other factors" mostly affect migraines headaches without aura. In the examined sample of adolescents suffering from headaches, 25.6% have migraine headache with aura, 67.2% have migraine headache without aura, and 7.25% have other migraine headaches, whereas in the group of adolescents with migraine headache indicating "other" factors as direct migraine headache triggers, 25.7% have migraine headache with aura, 73.3% have migraine headache without aura, and 1.0% have other migraine headaches. (Table 27. Effects of "other" triggering factors on migraine headache occurrence).

Lack of sleep as a trigger was equally reported in migraine headache and recurrent non-migraine headache (90, 6% vs. .94.5%). Particular food was indicated more often as a migraine headache trigger (72.4% vs. 32%; p<0.05). The most common dietary triggers implicated in migraine headache attacks were: meat (32.9%), eggs (30.5%) and aged cheese (27.7%). Odours were reported predominantly in migraine headaches, than in recurrent non-migraine headache (80.9 vs. 10%; p<0.05). Usual daily routine disturbance predominant in non-migraine headaches, was reported in migraine headaches and in of recurrent non-migraine headache (50.0% vs. 75.2%; p<0.05). Physical activity tends more often to trigger recurrent non-migraine headache than migraine headaches (85.3% vs. 45.3%; p<0.05). Tobacco smoking triggers similar migraine headaches and recurrent non-migraine headache (65% vs. 75%). Passive tobacco smoking triggers migraine headaches more often than recurrent non-migraine headache (81, 6% vs. 23.9%; p<0.05). The same is with alcohol drinking as a trigger (80, 2% vs. 68%; p<0.05). Psychical stress triggers equally recurrent non-migraine headache and migraine headaches (99.6% vs. 96, 9%). "Not eaten in time" was the trigger for 65% migraine headache attacks, whereas 32% of recurrent non-migraine headache (65% vs. 32%; p<0.05). Non-migraine headaches were, in general, more susceptible to weather changes than migraine headaches (78.8% vs. 21.28%) (p<0.05).

Table 28. **Migraine headache age dependent trigger factors.**

Trigger factor children with migraine // age groups (years)	10-11		12-13		14-15		16-17		SCORE	
	n	%	n	%	n	%	n	%	n	%
Lack of sleep	188	100	294	98.99	390	98.73	458	97.65	1330	98.6
Kinetosis	167	88.83	289	97.31	382	96.71	373	79.53	1211	89.8
Different food	145	77.13	252	84.85	380	96.20	425	90.62	1202	89.1
Psychic stress	71	37.77	239	80.47	393	99.49	469	100	1172	86.9
Odors	126	67.02	242	81.48	346	87.59	415	88.49	1119	82.9
Day activity disturbance	188	100	297	100	377	95.44	239	50.96	1101	81.62
Physical activity	164	87.23	246	82.83	322	81.52	273	58.21	1005	74.4
Passive tobacco smoke	126	67.02	194	65.32	201	50.89	178	37.95	699	51.8
Food deprivation	122	64.89	176	59.26	104	26.33	25	5.33	437	32.3
Other	64	43.04	83	27.95	87	22.02	53	11.30	287	21.28

Migraine: non-migraine headache; Lack of sleep – Pearson Chi Square: V 59610, DF 1, p<0.0001;
Kinetosis — Fisher Exact Test: V 735.350, DF 1, p<0.0001 ;
 Different food - Linear-by-Linear Association: V 1203.032, p<0.0001;
Chronic stress - Fisher Exact Test: V 94063. DF 2, p<0.0001;
Odor - Linear-by–Linear Association: V 1889.054, DF 1, p<0.0001;
Physical activity - Pearson Chi Square: V 69510, DF 1, p<0.0001;

Passive tobacco smoke - Fisher Exact Test: V 532.965, DF 1, p<0.0001;
Fatigue - Pearson Chi Square: V 55.445, DF 2, p<0.0001;
Psychological stress - Likelihood Ratio: V 1935.861, DF 1, p<0.0001;
Other - Pearson Chi Square: 2827.431, DF 1, p<0.0001

All of the trigger factors were age dependent. Trigger factors sensitivity in adolescent's migraine was stable during the adolescent age for "lack of sleep, odors, and weather changes". It increased for "different food and psychic stress", and decreased for "day activity disturbance and food deprivation" (Table 28-Migraine headache age dependent trigger factors).

Using Canonical Discriminate Analysis (coefficient over 0.3) migraine headaches were clearly distinguished from non-migraine headaches according to the headache triggers. The canonical discriminate coefficient was 0.77 for lack of sleep, 0.68 for passive tobacco smoking, 0.43 for odours, 0.58 for fasting, 0.45 for particular food, and borderline 0.336 for disturbance of daily routine activity (Table 29- Canonical discriminating analysis of migraine headache//non-migraine headache trigger factors in adolescents). They appeared as kinetosis, daily activity disturbance, food deprivation, and odors in younger adolescents (10-11 years old) and as odours, food type, and psychological stress in older adolescents (16-17 years old) without significant difference (Table 29. Age dependent canonical discriminating analysis of migraine headache//non-migraine headache trigger factors).

Table 29- Canonical discriminating analysis of migraine headache//non-migraine headache trigger factors in adolescents

Migraine trigger factors	Triggers reported in questionnaire %	Canonical discriminative analysis coefficient Migraine//non-migraine headaches
Psychical stress	96.9	-0.56
Lack of sleep	90.6	0.77
Tobacco passive smoke	81.6	0.68
Alcohol intake	80.2	0.63
Fasting	75.0	0.58
Odours	80.9	0.43
Tobacco smoke	72.3	0.43
Weather changes	78.8	-0.56
Specific type of food	72.4	0.45
Daily activity disturbance	50.0	0.336
Oversleeping	45.3	-0.38

Table 30-Age dependent canonical discriminating analysis of migraine headache//non-migraine headache trigger factors

Migraine trigger factors	Age groups (years)				
Migraine//non migraine headaches	10-11	12-13	14-15	16-17	SCORE
Daily activity disturbance	0.77	0.74	0.73	0.68	0.772
Lack of sleep	0.64	0.51	0.53	0.50	0.541
Odors	0.35	0.43	0.45	0.45	0.428
Foods	0.36	0.42	0.41	0.40	0.406
Fatigue	0.35	0.32	0.28	0.31	0.236
Psychological stress	0.22	0.18	0.28	0.36	0.216
Travel sickness (kinetosis)	0.36	0.43	0.10	0.09	0.159
Tobacco smoke	0.32	0.01	-0.10	-0.08	-0.081
Acute stress	-0.02	-0.02	-0.02	-0.15	-0.058
Food deprivation	-0.12	-0.04	0.03	0.02	-0.057
Oversleeping	-0.00	-0.01	-0.02	-0.05	-0.020

Discussion

Our study results are very similar to European Population Studies. Wober Bingol's (64). Population Study encountered prevalence of 3-17.6% of migraine headaches in adolescents. Describing pediatric headache, as a common health problem, Hershey found migraine in 10.6% of children between the age of 5 and 15 and in up to 28% of adolescents between the ages of 15 and 19 (65). Clear triggers as direct causes of migraine headache were occasionally proved in up to 10.4% of adolescents. They were highly significant for occurrence of migraine headache without aura. Chabriat H. et al., suggested that similar triggers could precipitate headache of different type (66).

The age of children and adolescents was of importance when identifying foods as direct triggers of migraine headaches. Some foods were indicated as direct triggers of migraine headache attacks (mean age 11 years and 8.9 months), whereas adolescents (mean age 10 years and 9 months), did not indicate food as a directtrigger of migraine attacks. They reported various odours as trigger factors of migraine headache attacks. This was in favor of slight, but still existing, higher susceptibility of younger perons to odours as trigger factors of migraine headache attacks, and vice versa in regard to foods.

Fatigue, mental stress, and lack of sleep are the main migraine headache triggers in most reports. There were three different combinations of sleep involvement, possibly due to more than one pathophysiological mechanism. Thirty percent of patients had migraine headache attack triggered by sleep; 24% by sleep deprivation and 6% by excess sleep. Sleep was also associated with the relief of migraine headache attacks. Oversleeping could not have been considered a trigger of headaches generally speaking. Although sleep problems were not a common complaint in migraine headache patients, the role of sleep habits and hygiene, as triggers of head pain, have been poorly analyzed. Bruni evaluated the effect of modifying bad sleeping habits across several headache parameters as very successful (67).

Apparently, there are trigger factors differentiating migraine headache from non-migraine headache but not vice versa. Identification of migraine headache trigger factors is extremely important in adolescents. Their elimination directly provides prevention of migraine headaches in adolescents. Typical migraine headache triggers in adolescents are lack of sleep, tobacco passive smoking, alcohol intakes, and "not eating at time". Based on the estimations of the most appropriate approach, up to 20% of headaches in general and up to 43% of migraine headache in adolescents might be preventable by removing risk factors amenable to intervention, with increasing proportions by age (68, 69).

We discussed only triggers that could be avoided (sleep disturbance, food, odours, tobacco smoke, alcohol drinks). During six months after migraine hedache reported 2.8 headaches per month, and 5.7 medications used during the month. Six months after strictly avoiding potential migraine headache trigger factors, adolescents reported 1.6 headaches per month and 2.4 medication used during the month. By avoiding recognized migraine headache trigger factors in our observed adolescent group, in 68% of adolescents 75% reduction of drugs used in headache therapy was achieved.

Conclusions and recommendations

It is extremely important to know all of the disposition factors of the adolescent's migraine headache. Recognizable during a period before migraine headache symptoms appear, they would enable its prevention by means of ultra-early prevention. Adequate prevention of migraine headaches should be initiated in the perinatal period and continued in each child with clearly predisposing factors for migraine syndrome.

Typical migraine headache triggers in adolescents are lack of sleep, tobacco passive smoking, alcohol intakes, and "not eating at time". All of migraine headache trigger factors are age dependent. Trigger factors are stable during the adolescent age for "lack of sleep, odors, and weather changes". During the adolescent age they increase for "different food and psychic stress", and decrees for "day activity disturbance, passive tobacco smoke, and food deprivation".

The prevalence of self-perceived triggers of headache does not correspond to the prevalence of identified risk factors for headaches. While the role of stress was overestimated, the high prevalence of the other confirmed risk factors in adolescents with headache suggests potential for prevention by increasing awareness for these risk factors and appropriate interventions. Identification of migraine headache trigger factors is extremely important in adolescents. Their elimination directly provides prevention of migraine headaches in adolescents.

Early detection of migraine headache trigger factors should be the prime concern not only of therapists, but also of parents whose children suffer from migraine headaches.

Literature

1. Merriam-Webster. "Adolescence". Retrieved May 9, 2012.

2. Macmillan Dictionary for Students Macmillan, Pan Ltd. 1981: 14-456. Retrieved 2010.7.15.

3. Dorn L. D, Biro F. M. "Puberty and Its Measurement: A Decade in Review. [Review]". Journal of Research on Adolescence. 2011;21(1):180–95.

4. Carlo G, Mestre M. V, McGinley M. M, Samper P, Tur., Sandman D. "The interplay of emotional instability, empathy, and coping on prosocial and aggressive behaviors". Personality and Individual Differences 2012;53(5):675–80.

5. Brown, B. Bradford; W. Larson, Reed; Saraswathi, T.S.; Nsamenang, A. Bame (2002). "3". The World's Youth: Adolescence in Eight Regions of the Globe. Cambridge University Press. p. 69. Retrieved 11 September 2014.

6. Knežević-Pogančev M. Cildren migraine syndrome definition and classification through time Medicinski pregled. 2008; 61(3-4):143-6.

7. Goadsby O, Olesen J. Diagnosis and management of migraine. BMJ 1996;312:1279-83.

8. Barlow CF. Headache and Migraine in Childhood. Clinics in Developmental Medicine. No 91 London S.I.M.P. with Blackwell Scientific; Philadelphia:1984.

9. Knežević-Pogančev M, Jović N, Filipović D, Ivetić V, Katanić D. Epidemiology and characteristics of migraine syndrome in children in Serbia. Neural Regen Res.2011;6(9):692-8.

10. Knežević Pogančev M. Migrenski sindrom dece. Zadužbina Andrejević. Todra, Beograd 2003.

11. Straube A, Heinen F, Ebinger F, von Kries R. Headache in school children: prevalence and risk factors. Dtsch Arztebl Int. 2013;110(48):811-8.

12. Kröner-Herwig B, Heinrich M, Morris L. Headache in German children and adolescents: a population-based epidemiological study. Cephalalgia. 2007 Jun;27(6):519-27.

13. Knežević-Pogančev M. Epidemiology, characteristics and distinctiveness of headaches in children from Vojvodina, Serbia. Neuroepidemiology. 2008;31(2):122-8.

14. Cvetkoić V, Plavec D, Hunjan-Lovrenčić A, et al. Prevalence and clinical characteristics of headache in adolescents: A Croatian epidemiological study Cephalalgia. 2014;34(4):289-97.

15. Abu-Arafeh I, Razak S., Sivaraman B, Graham C. Prevalence of headache and migraine in children and adolescents: a systematic review of population-based studies. Developmental Medicine & Child Neurology. 2010;52:1088–97.

16. Knežević-Pogančev M. "Specific features of migraine syndrome in children." The journal of headache and pain. 2006;7(4):206-10.

17. Fuh, J.L., Wang, S.-J., Lu, S.-R., Liao, Y.-C., Chen, S.-P. and Yang, C.-Y. Headache Disability Among Adolescents: A Student Population-Based Study. Headache: The Journal of Head and Face Pain. 2010;50:210–8.

18. Tonini M.C, Frediani F. Headache at high school: clinical characteristics and impact. Neurological Sciences. 2012;33(1):185-7.

19. Montagna P, Pierangeli G, Cortelli P. The Primary Headaches as a Reflection of Genetic Darwinian Adaptive Behavioral Responses. Headache: The Journal of Head and Face Pain. 2010;50:273–89.

20. Gargus JJ. Genetic Calcium Signaling Abnormalities in the Central Nervous System: Seizures, Migraine, and Autism. Annals of the New York Academy of Sciences. 2009;1151:133–56.

21. Lafrenière R. G. and Rouleau G. AIdentification of Novel Genes Involved in Migraine. Headache: The Journal of Head and Face Pain. 2012;52:107–10.

22. Bigal ME, Arruda MA. Migraine in the Pediatric Population—Evolving Concepts. Headache: The Journal of Head and Face Pain. 2010;50(7):1130–43.

23. Van Den Maagenberg AMJM, Terwindt GM, Haan J, Frants RR, Ferrari MD. Chapter 6 - Genetics of headaches. Handbook of Clinical Neurology. 2010;97:85-97.

24. Wöber-Bingöl C, Wöber C, Wagner-Ennsgraber C, Zebenholzer K, Vesely C, Geldner J, Karwautz A. IHS criteria and gender: a study on migraine and tension-type headache in children and adolescents. Cephalalgia. 1996;16(2):107-12.

25. Vahlquist B. Migraine in children. Int. Arch Allergy. 1955;7:348–55.

26. Bille B. A 40 year follow of school children with migraine. Cephalalgia. 1997;17940:488-91.

27. Hockaday JM. Headache in children. British Journal of Hospital Medicine. 1988;27:41-8.

28. Goadsby O, Olesen J. Diagnosis and management of migraine. BMJ. 1996; 312:1279-83.

29. Dalessio DJ. Diagnosing the severe headache. Neurology. 1994;44(3):6-12.

30. Michaele P, Henry P, Letenneuer L. Diagnosis screen for assessment of the IHS criteria for migraine by general practitioners. Cephalalgia. 1993;(12):54-9.

31. Mortimer MJ, Kay J.   A childhood migraine in general   practice clinical features and characteristics. Cephalalgia. 1992;12:238-43.

32. Fontanelle LM, et al. Migraine in childhood: difficulties in Diagnosis. Arh Neuropsichiatr. 1988;56(3B):553-8.

33. Headache Classification Committee of the International Headache Society (IHS). The International Classification of Headache Disorders 3rd edition (beta version) International Headache Society Cephalalgia. 2013;33(9)629–808.

34. Knežević-Pogančev M. Recurrent headache and migraine within the family. Genetika. 2011;43(1):101-12.

35. Russell M.B. Is migraine a genetic illness? The various forms of migraine share a common genetic cause Neurological Sciences. 2008;29(1)52-4.

36. Schürks M. "Genetics of migraine in the age of genome-wide association studies". The journal of headache and pain (Review) 2012;13(1):1–9.

37. Ducros A. Genetics of migraine. Revue neurologique. 2013;169(5):360–71.

38. Knežević-Pogančev M. Recurrent headache and migraine heritability - twin study. Genetika. 2011;43(3):595-606.

39. Stephen D. Silberstein MD, David W. Dodick MD. Migraine Genetics Part II Headache. 2013;53(8):1218-29.

40. Kröner-Herwig B, Jennifer Gassmann J, Headache Disorders in Children and Adolescents: Headache. 2012;52:1387-401.

41. AydinM, Kabakus N, Boydag S. Profile of children with migraine. The Indian Journal of Pediatrics 2010;77(11):1247-51.

42. Diklić V et al. Blood cerebrospinal fluid barrier impairment in vascular headaches Cephalagia. 1991;11:34-6.

43. Knežević-Pogančev M, Jović N, Doronjski-Bregun A, Šrek A, Filipović D. Breastfeeding duration influences migraine headache onset. Paediatr Croat. 2012;56(3):221-4.

44. Lehmann S, Milde-Busch A, Straube A, von Kries R, Heinen F. How specific are risk factors for headache in adolescents? Results from a cross-sectional study in Germany. Neuropediatrics. 2013;44(1):46-54.

45. Gargus J. J. Genetic Calcium Signaling Abnormalities in the Central Nervous System: Seizures, Migraine, and Autism. Annals of the New York Academy of Sciences. 2009;1151:133–56.

46. Montagna P., Pierangeli G. and Cortelli P. The Primary Headaches as a Reflection of Genetic Darwinian Adaptive Behavioral Responses. Headache: The Journal of Head and Face Pain. 2010;50: 273–89.

47. Wessman M, Terwindt G.M, Kaunisto M.A, Palotie A, Ophoff R.A. Migraine: a complex genetic disorder. Lancet Neurol. 2007;6(6):521-32.

48. Bigal M.E, Arruda M.A. Migraine in the Pediatric Population—Evolving Concepts Headache: The Journal of Head and Face Pain. 2010;50(7):1130–43.

49. Chakravarty A. How triggers trigger acute migraine attacks: a hypothesis. Med Hypotheses. 2010;74(4):750-3.

50. Milde-Busch A, Straube A, Florian Heinen F, R. Identified risk factors and adolescents' beliefs about triggers for headaches: results from a cross-sectional study J Headache Pain. 2012;13(8):639–43.

51. Lehmann S, Milde-Busch A, Straube A, von Kries R, Heinen F. How specific Are the Risk factors for Headache in Adolescents? Results from a Cross-sectional Study in Germany. Neuropediatrics. 2013;44:46-54.

52. Dorothée Neut, Antoine Fily, Jean-Christophe Cuvellier, and Louis Vallée. The prevalence of triggers in paediatric migraine: a questionnaire study in 102 children and adolescents J Headache Pain. 2012;13(1):61–5.

53. Knežević-Pogančev M, Jović N, Stojadinović A. Specific Triggers of Migraine Headache in Adolescents. Macedonian Journal of Medical Sciences. MJMS.1857-5773.2014.0435.

54. Annequin D, Tourniaire B. Migraine and headache in childhood. Arch Pediatr. 2005;12(5):624-9.

55. Spierings EL, Ranke AH, Honkoop PC. Precipitating and aggravating factors of migraine versus tension-type headache. Headache. 2001;41(6):554-58.

56. Mindell JA, Owens J, Alves R, Bruni O et al. Give children and adolescents the gift of a good night's sleep: a call to action. Sleep Med. 2011;12(30):203-4.

57. Milde-Busch A, Blaschek A, Heinen F, Borggräfe I, Koerte I, Straube A, Schankin C, von Kries R. Associations between stress and migraine and tension-type headache: results from a school-based study in adolescents from grammar schools in Germany. Cephalalgia. 2011;31(7):774-85.

58. Karli N, Zarifoglu M, Calisir N, Akgoz S. Comparison of pre-headache phases and trigger factors of migraine and episodic tension-type headache: do they share similar clinical pathophysiology? Cephalalgia. 2005;25(6):444-51.

59. Albers L, Milde-Busch A, Bazer O, Lehmann S, Riedel Ch, Bonfert M, Heinen F, Straube A and von Kries R. Prevention of Headache in Adolescents: Population-Attributable Risk Fraction for Risk Factors Amenable to Intervention. Neuropediatrics. 2013;44:40-45.

60. Milde-Busch A, Straube A, Heinen F, von Kries R. Identified risk factors and adolescents'beliefs about triggers for headaches: results from a cross-sectional study.J Headache Pain. 2012;13(8):639-43.

61. Headache Classification Committee of the International Headache Society. The International Classification of Headache Disorders;2nd edition. Cephalalgia.2004;24 (11):9-160.

62. Headache Classification Committee of the International Headache Society. The International Classification of Headache Disorders;2nd edition. Cephalalgia.2004;24 (11):9-160.

63. Olesen J. The International Classification of Headache Disorders, 2nd edition (ICHD-II) Rev Neurol (Paris).2005;16(6-7):689-91.

64. Wober–Bingol C, Wober C, Karwautz A. Diagnosis of headache in childhood and adolescence: a study of 437 patients Cephalalgia. 1993;13(13):207-37.

65. Hershey AD. What is the impact, prevalence, disability, and quality of life of pediatric headache? Curr Pain Headache Rep. 2005;9(5):341-4.

66. Chabriat H, Danchot J, Michel P, Joire JE, Henry P. Precipitating factors of headache. A prospective study in a national control-matched survey in migraineurs and nonmigraineurs. Headache. 1999;39(5):335-8.

67. Mindell JA, Owens J, Alves R, Bruni O et al. Give children and adolescents the gift of a good night's sleep: a call to action. Sleep Med. 2011;12(30):203-4.

68. Albers L, Milde-Busch A, Bayer O, Lehmann S, Riedel C, Bonfert M, Heinen F, Straube A, von Kries R. Prevention of headache in adolescents: population-attributable risk fraction for risk factors amenable to intervention. Neuropediatrics. 2013;44(1):40-5.

69. Martin PR. Managing headache triggers: think 'coping' not 'avoidance'. Cephalalgia. 2010; 30(5):634-7.

Definition of terms

Accompanying headache symptoms: symptoms that typically accompany rather than precede or follow headache. The most recognized migraine accompanying symptoms in adolescents are nausea, vomiting, photophobia, phonophobia, osmophobia, stomach pain and diarrhea.

Anorexia: lack of appetite and dislike for food. Anorexia in adolescents can be classified as mild, moderate or severe.

Aura: first symptom of an migraine headache attack in migraine with aura. Patophysiological migraine aura is the manifestation of focal cerebral dysfunction. The migraine headache aura typically lasts 20–30 minutes and precedes the headache.

Chronic adolescent headache pain : headache lasting through more days but not over a period longer than three months.

Close temporal relation: relation between an organic disorder and headache, usually known for disorders of acute onset where causation is likely, but not prouved.

Duration of headache: time from headache onset until headache termination.(A low-grade non-pulsating headache without accompanying symptoms may persist after migraine headache in adolescents, but it shell not ve included in migraine headache duration). If the adolescent falls asleep during an attack and wakes up relieved, migraine headache shall be considered as duration until time of awakening.

Facial pain: pain below the orbitomeatal line, above the neck and anterior to the pinnae.

Focal symptoms: ymptoms of focal brain (usually cerebral) disturbance such as occur in migraine aura.

Fortification spectrum: Angulated, arcuate and gradually enlarging visual hallucination typical of migrainous visual aura.

Frequency of migraine headache attacks: The rate of occurrence of attacks of migraine headache per time period. According to IHS Guidelines for Controlled Trials of Drugs in Migraine, 2nd edition (used in this book) it is recommended to caunt as migraine headache distinct attacks only separated by an entire day headache-free.

Headache: pain located above the orbitomeatal line.

Headache pain attack: headache pain that uilds up remains at a certain levetl for mminutes up to 72^h, and hten decrease until disapeares completely.

Intensity of pain: degree of pain expressed in terms of its functional consequence and scored at adolescent age on a verbal zero to five or zero to teen point scale. (Each adolescent has to choose degree of pain form absent to completely umposibility to do any ysuall activities).

Neuroimaging: CT (computerized tomography), MRI (magnetic resonance imaging), PET (positrone emission tomography) or scintigraphy of the brain.

New headache: any type, subtype or subform of headache from which the adolescent was not previously suffering.

Pain: an unpleasant sensory and emotional experience associated with actual or potential tissue damage, or described in terms of such damage.

Photophobia: hypersensitivity to light, usually causing avoidance.

Premonitory migraine headache symptoms: simptoms preceding and forewarning of a migraine attack by 2–48 hours, occurring before the aura in migraine with aura and before the onset of pain in migraine without aura. Moats common premonitory symptoms in migraine of adolescents are: fatigue, elation, depression, unusual hunger, craving for certain foods.

Prodrome: term which should be avoided, but previously has been used with different meanings, mostly synonymously with premonitory symptoms. Pulsating: Varying with the heart beat; throbbing.

Scintillation: Visual hallucinations that are bright and fluctuate in intensity, often at approximately 8–10 cycles/second. They are typical of migraine aura.

Scotoma: loss of part of the visual field of one or both eyes, with complete or relativeviion reduction.

Throbbing: synonym for pulsating.

Unilateral hedache: headache pain on either the right or the left side, not crossing the mid line, but not necessarily involving all of the right or left side of the head. Unilateral headache can be frontal, temporal or occipital only.

Vasospasm: constriction of artery or arterioles to such a degree that tissue perfusion is reduced.

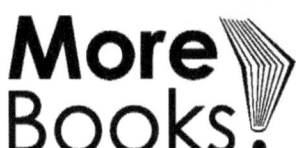

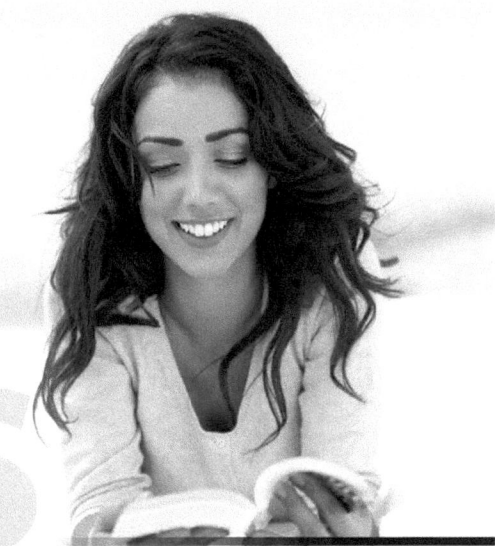

I **want** morebooks!

Buy your books fast and straightforward online - at one of the world's fastest growing online book stores! Environmentally sound due to Print-on-Demand technologies.

Buy your books online at

www.get-morebooks.com

Kaufen Sie Ihre Bücher schnell und unkompliziert online – auf einer der am schnellsten wachsenden Buchhandelsplattformen weltweit!
Dank Print-On-Demand umwelt- und ressourcenschonend produziert.

Bücher schneller online kaufen

www.morebooks.de

OmniScriptum Marketing DEU GmbH
Heinrich-Böcking-Str. 6-8
D - 66121 Saarbrücken
Telefax: +49 681 93 81 567-9

info@omniscriptum.com
www.omniscriptum.com

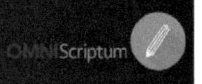

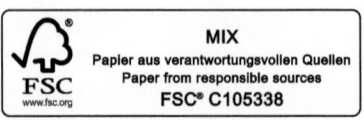

MIX
Papier aus verantwortungsvollen Quellen
Paper from responsible sources
FSC® C105338

Printed by Books on Demand GmbH, Norderstedt / Germany